I0478686

The Headache Pain Cure

How To Find Headache Pain Relief And Live A Happy Pain Free Life!

By
Michele Gilbert

<u>Visit My Amazon Author Page</u>

Dedicated to those who choose to stretch beyond their own limits and to seek a more abundant and fulfilling life

Your thoughts are creative.

Michele Gilbert

TABLE OF CONTENTS

My Free Gift to You!

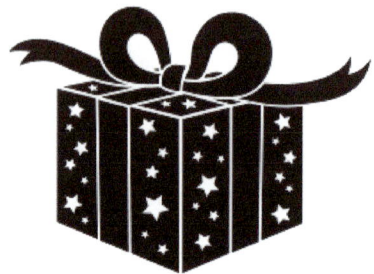

As a way of saying thank you for downloading my book, I am willing to give you access to a selected group of readers who (every week or so) receive inspiring, life-changing kindle books at deep discounts, and sometimes even absolutely free.

Wouldn't it be great to get amazing Kindle offers delivered directly to your inbox?

Wouldn't it be great to be the first to know when I'm releasing new fresh and above all sharply discounted content? Along with books on, Personal Development, and a variety of other great books.

But why would I so something like this?

Why would I offer my books at such a low price and even give them away for free when they took me countless hours to produce?

Simple Because I want to spread the word.

For a few short days Amazon allows Kindle authors to promote their newly released books by offering them deeply discounted (up to 70% price discounts and even for free. This allows us to spread the word extremely quickly allowing users to download thousands and thousands of copies in a very short period of time. Once the timeframe has passed, these books will revert back to their normal selling price.

That's precisely why you will benefit from being the first to know when they can be

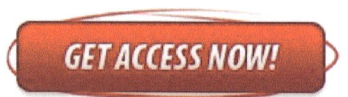

downloaded for Free!!!

So are you ready to claim your weekly Kindle books?

You are just one click away! Follow the link below and sign up to start receiving awesome content.

Thank you and Enjoy!

Introduction

I want to thank you and congratulate you for downloading the book, *"The Headache Pain Cure: How to Find Headache Pain Relief and Live a Happy Pain Free Life!"* This book contains proven steps and strategies on how to relieve the pain provoked by different types of headaches.

In this book we are offering detailed explanations on different causes and types of headaches and different approaches in treating the problem. We have offered some proven steps in relieving pain, but also preventing it from happening. Remember it is always better to try to prevent it than to cure it. If you have developed a chronic headache problem, this book will help you learn comprehensive ways in addressing your health problem and maintaining a healthy and active life.

Thanks again for downloading this book, I hope you enjoy it!

What are the causes and symptoms of headaches?

The head is one of the most common aching parts of the body. There are different types of headaches but one thing is sure, they are one of the most limiting types of soreness because they can block our everyday activities and duties. Because this condition is so widely spread doctors have constructed a classification for the types of headaches that help them address and treat the problem. The most types of headaches can be classified in three subcategories, primary, secondary and cranial neuralgias following by facial pain and other types of condition. Under these subcategories there are also different types of pain, so the primary headaches are differentiated into tension, migraine and cluster, in which the tension headaches are the most common type of the condition and are treated by over-the-counter medications for which a prescription is not needed. Tension headaches occur more frequently among women then man. 1 in 20 people in the world suffer from this type of the condition. Migraine headaches are the second typical form of the headaches. They affect children, as well as adults. Before puberty both sexes are affected equally, but after this period women are more likely to suffer from migraines. Primary headaches do affect significantly on the quality of the lifestyle. Secondary headaches represent a symptom on an injury or underlying illness so you should be careful about them. The structural problems range from infected teeth or sinus to meningitis or internal bleeding. If you experience headaches you should consult your doctor to be sure that there is not some deeper rooted reason of your health condition. There are some following symptoms that indicate the seriousness of the condition, so if you feel these sensations, you should contact your doctor immediately. These symptoms are: fever, stiff neck, and change in behavior, vomiting or weakness.

Headache is defined as a pain arising from the head or upper part of the neck. The pain is generated from the tissues surrounding the brain, because the brain is not neurologically structured to cause the sensation of pain, meaning that it has no nerves that give rise to the sensation of pain. The periosteum that surrounds bones; muscles surrounding the skull, sinuses, eyes, and ears; and meninges that cover the surface of the brain and spinal cord, arteries, veins, and nerves can become inflamed and cause a headache. There are different types of pain, ranging from dull constant sensation to sharp intense pain.

Tension headaches

Because the tension type of headache is most wide spread you will now learn what the symptoms of the condition are and get more detailed information about it. Common presentation of tension headaches are pain that begins in the back of the head and upper neck and includes the sensation of pressure, the most intense pressure is felt above the eyebrows. The pain can vary in intensity but it is usually not disabling, it does not prevent you for doing your day to day activities. The pain is not followed by any other bodily sensations as vomiting or audio/visual sensitivity. The appearance of the pain is sporadic and it is usually not frequent.

The causes of this type of headache are unknown. It is commonly thought, among the professionals, that the pain is caused by a contraction of muscles surrounding the skull. This type of headaches can occur due to the physical or emotional stress. Physical stress is caused by a hard and long term labor, or a job that requires long sitting hours, especially when the working on the computer is included.

If you think that you may suffer from tension headaches you should visit your doctor. The diagnosis is made by your health history. The person who is diagnosed with this condition usually complaints about mild or moderate aches, located on both sides of the head. Tension headache sufferers do not notice the worsening of the pain with the increase of the activity. Still, even though tension headaches are not life threatening, daily activities could become more difficult to accomplish.

Drug treatment of headaches

In this book you will learn the ways in treating the primary type of headaches, mostly tension headaches. As we have mentioned, some over the counter drugs are most commonly used in relieving the tension headache pain, such as aspirin, ibuprofen, acetaminophen and naproxen. When using these drugs you should keep some things in mind. Aspirin should not be used in children younger than 14 years of age, because this drug can be a trigger in developing Reye`s syndrome, a life threatening neurological condition. People are usually not careful with this drug because it is most common used in different type of conditions and for different aches to be relieved. There are some serious side effects that can occur when using the drug, such as gastrointestinal bleeding, heartburn, ulcers and anaphylaxis, a life threatening allergic reaction. Ibuprofen is known for the possibility of causing gastrointestinal bleeding, nausea, rash, liver damage and gastrointestinal upset. Acetaminophen seems as the least harmful of the commonly used drugs. There is still risk of developing changes in blood and liver damage. Naproxen is known for having similar side effects as ibuprofen, including vomiting, rash and liver damage. There are also some other pain relievers that are prescribed if the person is experiencing headache, such as fenoprofen, flubiprofen, nabumetone etc. These pain relief meds are usually safe when used as directed, but, besides the side effects you should keep these facts in mind.

- Get informed about the active ingredients in every medicine to be sure if you are allowed to use the meds. Maybe you are allergic to some ingredient. Read the label thoroughly and carefully.
- Never exceed the recommended dosage on the package
- Take care of the way you are using this type of drugs, it is easy to over-medicate yourself.
- You should ask your doctor for approval before using the meds that contain aspirin, ibuprofen or naproxen, especially if you have a bleeding

problem, asthma, if you have underwent any type of surgery recently or you are about to have one. You should also ask for advice if you have ulcers, any type of kidney or liver disorder.

When using pain relief drugs avoid excessive caffeine usage and mixing it with other over-the-counter meds. Any medication containing barbiturates or narcotics should be used sparingly. If you notice that you are using the meds more than twice a week, you should visit a doctor who will prescribe you a headache therapy. Overuse of symptomatic pain relief drugs can cause more frequent headaches and resistance to the medication.

Biofeedback therapy

There are some automatic functions in our body that occur without us being aware of them. Breathing is the best example of these processes and functions, because we are not aware that we are breathing, we do it naturally without thinking about it. Biofeedback is a way of gaining control over these processes in order to achieve a more relaxed state of your organism. You will learn more about your automatic bodily activities, which will help you in controlling the functions of your body and also in relieving the pain. Biofeedback is a practice that involves learning how your body functions and learning how to control it.

There are different types of biofeedback therapy. EMG biofeedback is based on the muscle tension control, while on the other hand thermal biofeedback and blood flow feedback relate to the information regarding blood flow. Never mind which type of biofeedback therapy you choose it will all begin the same way. Individual is hooked up to a computer that shows the physiology of one's body. According to specialist thermal biofeedback is the most effective in treating the headaches. A person suffering from headaches will learn how to monitor the severity of the pain, or even prevent it, if using the therapy 20-30 minutes, 2-3 times a week.

Biofeedback therapy is especially effective when combined with relaxation techniques. These techniques are based to teach you how to achieve a physical and mental state of calm and relaxation. You sure do have some activities that you find relaxing, but, relaxation techniques are actually a systematic set of activities that you have to learn in order to apply them right. Relaxation procedures are crucial in curing primary type of headaches, because, as we have mentioned, they are in most cases caused by a stressful everyday life. Relaxation training and techniques slow down the sympathetic nervous system which is responsible for stress response.

There are different relaxation techniques that you can use for achieving your emotional and physical balance. One of which is the deep breathing technique.

You should place one hand on your chest and one on your abdomen to be aware of the breathing process. Afterwards you should breathe in through your nose and exhale through the mouth, very slowly. Whilst breathing try to pull your breath towards your belly, and feel it filling with air. This process you will have to practice to get the best results. But once you have learned it, it will help you to maintain the emotional calm, much needed for avoiding stress that can trigger your headaches. Besides deep breathing there are progressive muscle relaxation and many different relaxation techniques, that you can be thought by a professional if you want to try them out. Remember, it is always better to avoid chemical treatment in favor of alternative ways of relieving pain. A stress and pain free life is what you want to achieve, and this could be done by a regular practice and techniques that would do you good.

Exercises that will relieve your pain

Besides the generally healthy way of life, enough sleep, avoiding stress etc., there are some exercises that could help you prevent headaches. These exercises take 15-20 minutes a day, but are effective in reducing the risk of developing headache condition and attacks of pain. **Gentle neck and shoulder exercises may be used to relax and stretch strained, shortened muscles.** This can reduce tension and decrease the risk of headaches triggered by muscle tension. These exercises that you will now have a chance to learn are equally effective for tension headache sufferers and migraine sufferers.

- **Neck rotation -** Rotate your head till you look straight out over one shoulder, all the way keeping your head in the same level. When you reach the point, stay in this position for 10-20 minutes, and look down at your shoulder. Return your head to a starting position, and do the same other way around.

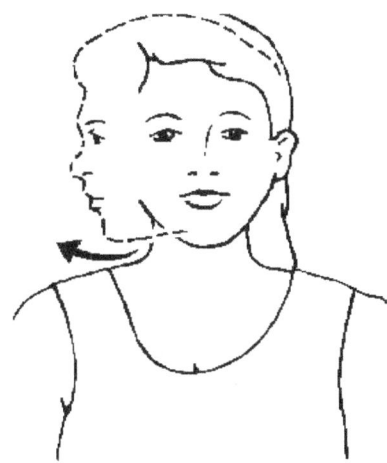

- **Neck retraction** - Squeeze your shoulder blades together and whilst in this position pull your head straight back, keeping in mind to keep it level. Stay in this position for 10 seconds and get to the starting position. Repeat this movement 10 times. Remember do it slowly, you should not feel any pain.

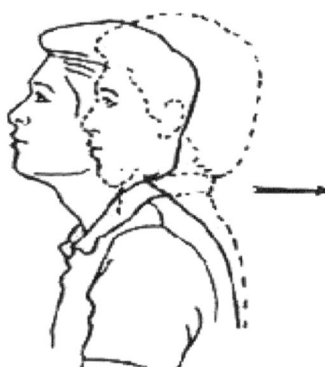

- **Chinning** - The starting position is the same as in previous two exercises place your head in its natural level and look straight ahead, then inhale and tuck in your chin. Afterword exhale and stick out your chin. You should repeat this movement 3-5 times, and remember to breathe. This exercise helps strengthening your neck muscles and keeping your head in a right position.

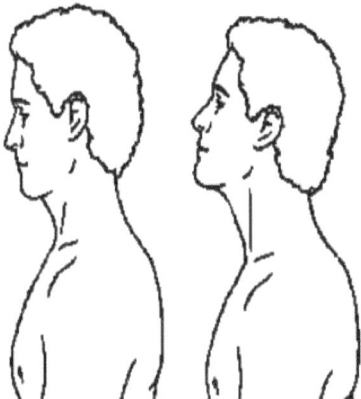

- **Shoulder shrug** - Keep your arms relaxed by your body. Lift your shoulders towards your ears. Squeeze your shoulder blades and rotate your shoulders to the back and then down to the starting position. Repeat this exercise 10 times. You should keep in mind that you should never rotate your shoulders forwards.

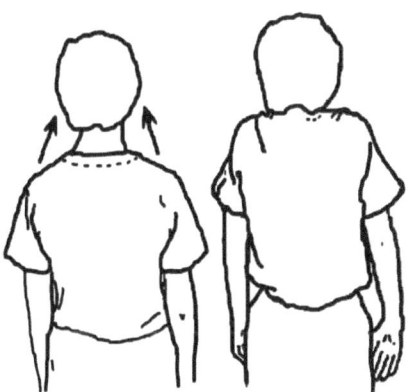

- **Shoulders retraction** - Touch your fingers to your ears and slightly raise your elbows. All the time remember not to push or pull on the neck. Squeeze your shoulder blades together. Stay in this position for 5 seconds and then release.

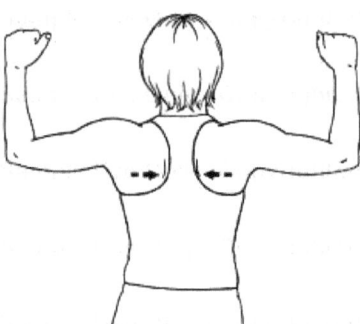

- **Upper back stretch.** Extend your arms in front of your body, clasp your hands together. Pull your shoulder blades apart gently, and then drop your chin to your chest. Hold this position for 10-30 seconds. Repeat this movement 10 times.

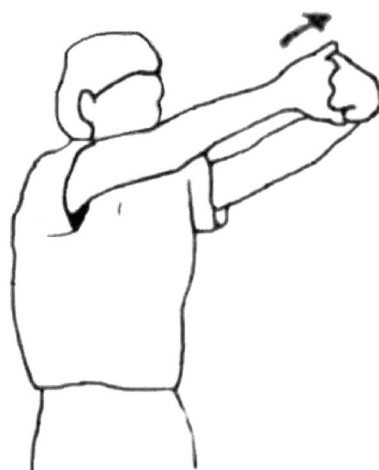

Neck muscles that run from the upper and middle neck down to the lower neck and shoulder blades are usually the initial cause of tension headaches, and stretching them will help you reduce the pain and keep your head pain free. If you feel that you would benefit more from customized exercises you should ask your doctor for tips or physical therapy.

Like with any other type of exercises you should remember to stay consistent and stick to your routine. These exercises will take 10-20 minutes of your daily free time, but in return you will live a life without constant headaches which tire and frustrate you.

Diet for preventing headaches

Research has shown that there are some proven ways in preventing the headaches by adjusting your diet plan. Vitamin b2 is one of the headache killers; it reduces the problem for up to 50%. This ingredient improves your brain metabolism and its muscles cells, which helps the brain in maintaining the much needed energy. Food rich in b2 is for example crimini mushrooms or asparagus, or to keep it simple a glass of low-fat milk. There are also diet supplements containing vitamin b2.

It is mentioned that women suffer from headaches more often than man. It is believed that the estrogen level can trigger this condition. In this case magnesium is helpful if you experience headaches on monthly basis. Try to add 450 mg of magnesium to your daily diet. Spinach is a rich source of this element, also Swiss chard. Besides this two there are some more foods containing magnesium, but in smaller amounts, such as sweet potatoes, bananas, sunflower seeds and sesame seeds.

You should add coenzyme Q10 which you can find in mackerel and tuna, broccoli and cauliflower. To get the best results be sure to get at least 100 mg of Q10 on the daily basis. This coenzyme is a rich source of energy production and therefore it is important for keeping your blood vessels healthy. Besides, it is a very powerful antioxidant. By eating food rich with this coenzyme you will protect your body from stress-induced free radicals.

While this as a basis for your new headache killer diet you should only add water-rich fruit like watermelon, strawberries, grapefruit or pineapple. Remember to stay hydrated, because it is very important to maintain the water balance in your organism. Also, you should remember to avoid smoking, exaggerating with alcohol and caffeine. There are some foods that are proven to affect the severity of headaches, so you should try to minimize the usage of this food in your every day nutrition plan. Those are: dairy, chocolate, peanut butter, fruits such as avocado and banana, meat with nitrates, such as hot dogs and bacon, basically any over processed food.

Homeopathic treatment

In this part you will learn how to treat your headaches naturally, by home-made homeopathic remedies. There are some herbs and cures that were proven successful in addressing the problem of headaches and migraines. If you want to treat your condition avoiding chemical treatment then you should try out these natural cures that do not have side effects and can significantly improve your overall health status.

- **Lavender Oil.** Lavender oil is known for its great impact on health and different condition. The herb smells great and what is most important it is proven that lavender oil can reduce headaches. You can inhale it or apply it topically, that is on you to decide which way suits your needs best. If you choose to inhale the herb, pour 2-3 drops of the oil in the same amount of cups of boiling water. You should inhale the evaporating water, whilst covered by a towel, or something similar. Unlike other medical oils, you can apply it directly to your skin without diluting it. It is not recommended to use the herb orally.
- **Peppermint Oil.** Peppermint is a soothing home remedy that has been shown to benefit avoiding different types of headaches, especially tension headaches. This has a vaso-constricting and vaso-dilating properties, which helps in controlling a healthy blood flow through your organism. We have mentioned before that headaches can appear as a result of a poor blood flow. It is now clear how the peppermint oil has a great impact on this types of headaches. Also, because of the sharp smell, this oil opens up the sinuses. Corked sinuses are often a reason for headaches, so opening them up is a crucial step in treating this type of headaches.
- **Basil oil.** Basil is a great choice for tension headaches because it works as a muscle relaxant. Exercises that help you relax your tense muscles in combination with this oil are a great home remedy. You can use the oil to massage the stiff areas of your neck in order to relax.

- **Feverfew -** Feverfew is used to reduce the bodily temperature, but it is also good in helping to relieve headaches. There are studies that prove that feverfew is best to be taken on daily basis, especially in combination with white willow, which contains properties similar to aspirin, but without any harmful side effects.
- **Flaxseed -** Omega 3 fatty acids, stored in flaxseed, can reduce headaches provoked by different types of inflammation processes. You can use it in different forms, ranging from oil to whole seed.
- **Apple cider vinegar**. This ingredient has a long history as a successful natural remedy. It's been used to relieve everything from scurvy to hay fever. Some modern day studies have proven its effectiveness in treating certain illnesses, but most of its clout lies in the reports of people throughout the centuries who have benefited from it. This remedy will help improving your circulation and you will benefit a lot from it. Try to drink it with water every morning and you will notice the results in improving your overall health, but especially headaches.

Besides this most used remedies there are a lot of other cures that you can try out, for example cayenne pepper, fish oil, gingerroot etc. Basically anything that helps your blood flow and that helps you relax will be a useful way in treating your problem.

Remember living a healthy life and changing of your everyday habits is a successful key in getting rid of headaches, or any other problem of modern man living in a stressful society. Sleep enough, eat healthy, exercise and avoid chemical treatment, unless you really have to use it. With a more relaxed point of view, and caring for your body it is guaranteed you will achieve great results in maintaining a healthy and active life long into future.

Conclusion

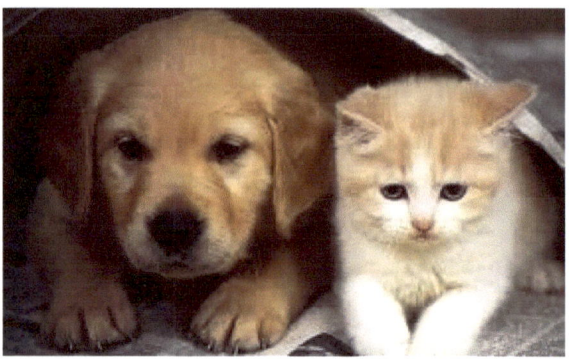

Before you go, I'd like to say thank you for purchasing my book.

I know you could have picked so many other books to read on treating headache pain.. But you took a chance on me.

So A Big thanks for downloading this book and reading it all the way to completion.

Now I would like to ask a _small_ favor.

Could you please take a minute or two to leave a review for this book on Amazon?

Click here

The feedback will help me continue to publish more kindle books that will help people to get better results in their lives.

And if you found it helpful in anyway then please let me know :-)

Preview of My New Book.
Help! I'm In Love With A Narcissist

So There's This Person...

So you've met this person who seems to have it all together, it all figured out, and the cat's in the bag. They're the kind of person who steps into the room with the presence of a floodlight and when they leave, it feels like they took the oxygen with them. They're captivated by all the boring stuff you've crammed into your calendars and call a life, but more importantly, they make you feel great. Every word you say is scooped up and filed away in their brains because they're actively engaging with you. They're making you feel like you're the only person in the room.

I mean, they're dedicated to themselves. They've been grooming themselves impeccably, or maybe they've moved beyond that. Maybe they've transcended the need to look good and they're just all about their intellectual prowess that they're willing to share with you—YOU, mere mortal! This person is the one person you know that could sell snow to an Inuit.

Sure, they might talk like they're trying to sell you something, or you might get the chills when you shake their hand, but come on, they're really great! They're a riot to be around and there's no way that you're just going to give up on hanging out with someone this cool.

But after a while, it might grate against you. After all, you watch as they move from one person to the next at parties, dancing around like the social butterfly that they are. It might start out as jealousy that you're not getting the majority of their time. It might bother you that all that special treatment that they gave you is just their average operating mode, which they treat everyone incredible, regardless of whom they are or what their lives are like. But after a moment, the jealousy is going to fade, because there's a truth hiding in there that is just nagging at you—clawing at you—to get out.

This might be because you're picking up on something no quite right about them. It means that you might be picking up on a subtle reality that's lurking behind those charming eyes and that million dollar smile that's starting to rub you the wrong way more and more. It's something more and most likely, you're picking up on the fact that the person you're bothered by might be a narcissist.

Of course, there are Narcissists and there are narcissists. A subtle difference in writing that makes all the difference and we're going to talk about both of them in this book. There are people out there that are really full of themselves. They're people who make life difficult for themselves and for those that are working with them and there are ways for us as regular people to deal with them. There are ways around them and there are ways to truly identify them.

After all, you don't want to peg Cool Jim as a Narcissist when he just has an over inflated ego. So where do you start? Well, reading this book was a great decision, because we're going to figure out together if Cool Jim is really someone you should be avoiding or if this is someone that you should just try your hardest to ignore and maybe just avoid at parties. In the end, we're going to find out what it is that you're dealing with.

So, want to go hunting for a narcissist? Or is it a Narcissist?

O Muses

So, once upon a time, the Greeks decided that there was a story that needed to be told. It was the tale of how a river god and a nymph decided to get together for a little tryst that resulted in the birth of an exceptionally beautiful young man you was declared as Narcissus. Now, this wasn't a man who was just 90's Brad Pitt gorgeous, but the male version of Helen of Troy. He drove the ladies and the men crazy. People wanted him and they wanted to be him. There's something about this guy that really made people go wild. They wanted him and when you're a hot commodity, demand tends to turn to worship and worship does something nasty for the people who aren't ready for it.

Narcissus had a commodity that was in high demand. That means that people were all over him and the desire for him is what inevitably drove Narcissus to a dark, cold place that made him resentful and spiteful of those that loved and desired him. As they flocked to him, Narcissus became a tool and a douche. He was rude and mean and cruel to everyone that came after him. In essence, he came to believe exactly what they told him he was a little too much.

Seeing this, the goddess of revenge decided that it was time to bring him down to reality after his cruelty and rudeness toward others. So while Narcissus was out hunting all manly and such, he came across an enchanted pool that the goddess of revenge made just for him. Well, when Narcissus found the pool, he gazed into it and found his reflection and fell in love with it. For the first time in his life, Narcissus found in love with someone, only that it's himself. Gazing into the pool, night and day passed as he gazed at the reflection in the pool.

Then, before anyone can tell him what an idiot he's being, his selfish love is rewarded with him falling into the pool and drowning because he couldn't take his eyes off himself.

There's a lot that can be taken away from this story and there's a lot that is freakishly familiar with what's going to follow in these next few chapters. So there's this happy little moment at the end of this chapter that I get to tell you why this story is important and it's going to be great. So here you go:

Click Here To Read The Rest Of
Help! I'm In Love With A Narcissist

P.S. You'll find many more books like this and others under my name Michele Gilbert.

Don't miss them… here is a short list.

Wicca: The Ultimate Beginners Guide For Witches and Warlocks: Learn Wicca Magic

The Introvert's Advantage: The Introverts Guide To Succeeding In An Extrovert World

Stop Playing Mind Games: How To Free Yourself Of Controlling And Manipulating Relationships

Instant Charisma: A Quick And Easy Guide To Talk, Impress, And Make Anyone Like You

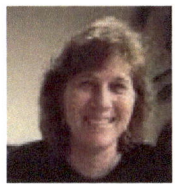

Michele Gilbert was born and raised in Brooklyn, New York. Drawn to literature and writing at a young age, she enrolled at Brooklyn College and majored in English. After graduation Michele did not begin writing immediately, instead she embarked on a career in the finance industry and spent the next thirty years on Wall Street.

Serendipity struck when she least expected it. After ending a long-term relationship, Michele found herself lost and unsure what the future held. She began to read books on grief and loss, looking for answers. Those led her to delve deeper into the Law of Attraction and its power. What resulted was remarkable. Not only had she begun to heal, she had also rekindled her former love of writing and discovered her life's purpose.

The years have taken her through many twists and turns, but she learned valuable lessons along the way. Today she publishes books-mostly self-help and metaphysical in nature-and feels compelled to share her knowledge with those facing similar experiences. Her greatest hope is to inspire others and show them ways to overcome adversity and gracefully accept life's inevitable low points.

Going forward, she plans to incorporate more teachings of self-help, finance and meditation. Regular meditation is very beneficial to her progress as she forges a new life. Morning rituals and positive incantations are other practices Michele embraces; they are very restorative in daily life.

As an avid hiker, Michele and fellow club members often hike the picturesque Jersey Pine Barrens. She is a history buff, voracious reader, baseball fanatic and a foodie. She also proudly supports Trout Unlimited-a national non-profit organization dedicated to conserving, protecting and restoring North America's Coldwater fisheries and their watersheds.

Michele currently resides forty minutes from Atlantic City and the Jersey Shore. She makes her home with a Blue Russian rescue cat named Jersey, though she isn't exactly sure who rescued who.

Michele really enjoys publishing books that can make a difference in people's lives. If you have any suggestions or would like to have a specific topic covered in a future book, please send an email to michelegilbertbooks@gmail.com and we will get back to you.

Thanks for reading!

www.ingramcontent.com/pod-product-compliance
Lightning Source LLC
Chambersburg PA
CBHW041615180526
45159CB00002BC/860